Sayed Md. Samser Nahid

Outcome of Different Modalities Treatment of Sigmoid Volvulus

Pradip Kumar Nath
AZM Mostaque Hossain
Sayed Md. Samser Nahid

Outcome of Different Modalities Treatment of Sigmoid Volvulus

LAP LAMBERT Academic Publishing

Imprint

Any brand names and product names mentioned in this book are subject to trademark, brand or patent protection and are trademarks or registered trademarks of their respective holders. The use of brand names, product names, common names, trade names, product descriptions etc. even without a particular marking in this work is in no way to be construed to mean that such names may be regarded as unrestricted in respect of trademark and brand protection legislation and could thus be used by anyone.

Cover image: www.ingimage.com

Publisher:
LAP LAMBERT Academic Publishing
is a trademark of
International Book Market Service Ltd., member of OmniScriptum Publishing Group
17 Meldrum Street, Beau Bassin 71504, Mauritius

Printed at: see last page
ISBN: 978-613-9-95341-7

Zugl. / Approved by: Dhaka, Dhaka Medical College Hospital, Diss.,2013

Outcome of Different Modalities Treatment of Sigmoid Volvulus; A Study of 50 cases.

Dr. Pradip Kumar Nath

GUIDED BY

Professor AZM Mostaque Hossain
Head of the department
Dhaka Medical College
Dhaka, Bangladesh

Abstract

Background

The treatment of sigmoid volvulus is a complex procedure. Many studies have shown that patient with early presentation where laparoscopic intervention can be done, the outcome is better. The currently accepted surgical procedures for sigmoid volvulus include resection with primary anastomosis or resection and Hartman procedure. Primary anastomosis is performed if the divided bowel ends are viable, peritoneal contamination is not evident, and the patient is hemodynamically stable. The other methods are Paul-Mikulicz procedure, sigmoidopexy, mesosigmoidoplasty, extraperitonealization of sigmoid colon, mesenteropexy, laparoscopic fixation and percutaneous endoscopic colopexy usingcolonscopy. The aim of this study is to determine the various outcome of various methods sigmoid volvulus and to search for a relatively safe, easy and economic protocol which can be adopted in Bangladesh.

Objectives:

- To observe the outcome of sigmoid volvulus treatment in different methods.
- To find out a safe protocol for management of sigmoid volvulus which can be adopted in our country.

Study design:

Descriptive case series

Study setting and period

General surgery wards of Dhaka Medical College Hospital, Dhaka for a period of six months from July 2012 to December 2012.

Patients

Fifty patients who admitted with intestinal obstruction due to the volvulus of sigmoid colon in surgery department during study period were included in this study by consecutive sampling.

Method

At enrollment particulars of patients were recorded. Preoperative investigations, proper resuscitation, nasogastric tube, indwelling catheter,antibiotics and analgesics were given according to the standardized protocol. Decision was made for procedure of decompression of colon. Primary anastomosis of colon or exteriorization depends upon the condition of the gut and confidence as well as expertise of the surgeon. At every postoperative follow up patients were observed for time to first bowel movement postoperatively,postoperative complications like vomiting, abdominal distension, anastomotic leakage, febrile illness, wound infection. Length of hospital stay, routine follow after four weeks was recorded. All data were recorded in a prescribed case record form. At the end of the study data were analyzed and the results were submitted.

Main outcome measures
i.   Treatment measures or what type of operation was performed.
ii. Time to first oral intake.
iii. Postoperative ileus.
iv. Wound complications.
v.   Anastomotic leakage.
vi. Revisional surgery.
vii. Death

Result

Fifty patients were included in the study. Thirty eight (76%) patients were males and twelve (24%) patients were females. Male to Female ratio was 3.17: 1. Age ranged from 20 years to 70 years. The mean age was 54.98years (SD $\pm$ 11.27). Almost all patient (100%) presented with abdominal distention and failure to pass stool or flatus. 74% patients suffered from colicky abdominal pain. Commonlyperformed operation procedure was Hartmann's operation 21patients (42%). Resection and primary anastomosis was done on 16 patients (32%), Resection and primary anastomosis with proximal diversion on 7 patients (14%) and Resection with double barrel colostomy on 6 patients (12%). During operation 100% gut edema was found whereas gangrene was found in 30% and perforation in 16%. Mean operation time was 2.43 (SD $\pm$ 0.25) hours. Bowel moved within 48 to 72 hours in 52% patient. Postoperative complications were observed upto to the discharge of the patient. Postoperativecomplication as well as death rate was low in Resection and Primary anastomosis.

Conclusion

Resection and Primary anastomosis could be the most convenient and economic operative procedure which also ensured lower morbidity rate of the patient.

Keywords: Sigmoid volvulus, Resection, anastomosis, colostomy.

Table of Contents

List of Tables

List of figures

XI

ACKNOWLEDGEMENT

It is a great pleasure to express my deep gratitude, due respect and profound indebtedness to **Professor Dr. A Z M Mostaque Hossain,** FCPS (Surgery), Professor of Surgery, Dhaka Medical College and Hospital. I am very much grateful for his continuous supervision and guidance on every aspect of the study, which helped me for the successful accomplishment of the task.

I am also highly grateful to Prof. Dr.Hasan Md. AbdurRouf (Surgery-CMC),Prof. Dr. Md. ShahidHossain (Surgery-DMC), Prof.Dr.Md.Faruk Ahmad (Surgery-CoMC), Prof. Dr. A B M KhurshidAlam (Surgery-CoMC), Prof. Dr. Md.SerajulHoque (Urology-CoMC), Dr. A B M Jamal(Asso Prof. Of Surgery-DMC), Dr. Syed Anwaruzzaman (Asst. Prof of Ortho Syrgery-CoMC), Dr. Jahangir HossainBhuiyan (Asst Prof Of Surgery-CoMC) for their valuable suggestions and comments.

 I am thankful to my colleaguesDr.A H M AfzalulHoque, Dr.A Z MahmudulHasan, Dr. Moinul Islam, Dr. Abdullah Md.Abu AyubAnsary, Dr. NiazurRahman for their kind help in collecting materials for the study.

Last but not the least, I am very much grateful to those patient who gave consent to be sample of this study, without whose participation it would not be possible to conduct this study.

(Dr.Pradip Kumar Nath)

Chapter: One
Introduction

Introduction

Volvulus is defined as an abnormal twisting of a segment of bowel on itself, along its longitudinal axis. This results in occlusion of the proximal bowel and a closed loop obstruction within the segment[1]. Compromised blood supply to the involved segment, together with the increase in intraluminal pressure, leads to gangrene and perforation if obstruction is unrelieved.

Worldwide, the incidence of volvulus of the large bowel varies widely. In an advanced westernpopulationvolvulus accounts for 1-5% of all large bowel obstructions. In these populations, the most common site of large bowel torsion is the sigmoid colon (80%), followed by cecum (15%) transverse colon (3%) and splenic flexure (2%). In the "volvulus belt" of Africa and the Middle East, 50% of large bowel obstructions are a result of volvulus, almost exclusively of the sigmoid colon. In Northern Iran, sigmoid volvulus accounts for 85% of large bowel obstructions.

In the vast majority of cases, sigmoid volvulus is an acquired condition, resulting from elongation of the sigmoid loop and stretching of the sigmoid mesocolon. This is in contrast to cecal volvulus, which results most commonly from failure of retroperitoneal fixation of the cecum[2].

Volvulus of the sigmoid colon occurs in the face of the following conditions; 1) Band of adhesions (peridiverticulitis) 2) Overloaded pelvic colon 3) Long pelvic mesocolon 4) Narrow attachment of pelvic mesocolon 5) Idiopathic megacolon, which initiates the torsion process[4].

The volvulus patient is often debilitated and bedridden. Because of the frequent association with neurologic or psychiatric impairment, a reliable history is often not available. The patient, or their attendant, may give a history of previous episodes of abdominal pain and distension, with the inability to pass flatus. An unknown proportion of these episodes of volvulus are self limiting. With each episode of volvulus, the base of the mesocolon becomes increasingly narrow and therefore predisposed to recurrent bouts. Abdominal distension is frequently massive and characteristically tympanitic over the gas-filled, thin-walled sigmoid loop. Overlying tenderness or peritonism raises the concern of ischemic or perforated bowel. Depending on the extent of ischemia or leakage, systemic toxicity may be apparent[2].

Diagnosis of sigmoid volvulus is usually obvious from a plain abdominal radiograph, which shows the characteristic "omega" or "inverted loop" sign. In doubtful cases a limited Gastrografin enema will reveal the characteristic "beaked" appearance of the apex of the volvulus in the distal sigmoid[3].

The first priority is resuscitation of the patient. This should be performed in a well staffed facility which is equipped for X-rays, invasive monitoring and rigid sigmoidoscopy. Vomiting and third space fluid loss into the sigmoid colon results in hypovolemic shock which must be corrected with intravenous balanced salt solutions such as Ringer's Lactate. Fluid resuscitation should be initiated before any attempts are made to reduce the volvulus. In the event of inadvertent perforation, the patient will be more adequately perfused and any further delay to optimize the patient's general condition before surgery will be minimized.

Hypovolemic shock may be compounded by sepsis in the presence of ischemic bowel. For the same reasons given above, broad spectrum antibiotics (aerobic and anaerobic) should be given to pre-empt a sigmoidoscopic perforation. The patient is laid in the left lateral position to improve venous return which may be compromised as a result of massive abdominal distension. Oxygen is given, since splinting of the diaphragm impedes respiratory efforts and results in "shunting" of blood through the pulmonary circulation. A foley catheter is inserted to assess fluid balance and a nasogastric tube should be placed if vomiting is a prominent symptom or X-ray reveals significant small bowel obstruction.

Emergency surgery is the definitive treatment of sigmoid volvulus if there is any evidence of bowel ischemia or peritonitis or failure of endoscopic decompression. Conversely, if the patient has neither of the above and endoscopic decompression and detorsion are successful, semi-elective surgery during the same hospital stay is acceptable. Bowel decompression is continued via a rectal tube while the bowel is prepared and the patient stabilized[5].

The treatment of sigmoid volvulus has evolved over the past decades from one requiring immediate surgical correction, which carries a high mortality, to one of immediate sigmoidoscopic decompression and elective surgery with its attendant lower mortality. Even from the time of Hippocrates, decompression of the volvulus was attempted using a long suppository "10 digits long" into the rectum. This mode of deflating the volvulus was suggested again in 1859 by Gay in England, but did not gain widespread acceptance until the middle of the next century.

Open reduction of the volvulus at laparotomy was first described by Atherton in 1883, although recurrence rates were high and fixation or resection of the sigmoid was attempted. Emergency resection carried a mortality rate of well over 50%, and sigmiodopexy was found to have a high rate of recurrence[4].

The failure of sigmiodpexy was illustrated during re-exploration of the abdomen for recurrent volvulus, which often revealed little evidence of the attempted fixation. In 1947

Bruusgaard revived the technique of transanal deflation using sigmoidoscopy. Sigmoidoscopic decompression gained widespread acceptance due to high mortalities in urgent laparotomy. More recently the use of the flexible sigmoidoscope or colonoscope provides a further weapon in the armamentarium of the surgeon attempting nonoperative reduction of the sigmoid loop[2].

The recent advancement in laparoscopic surgery provides another dimension to the evolving treatment of sigmoid volvulus. Although laparoscopic intervention, in its current mode, will not play a role in reduction of the acute volvulus, its use in elective resection of the redundant sigmoid loop may be facilitated by anatomic considerations. The mobile nature of the sigmoid loop itself may also facilitate its mobilization and reduce the risk of damage to adjacent structures. Lastly, the close apposition of the proximal rectum and distal left colon (as a result of the shortened mesosigmoid) may facilitate the performance of a stapled end-to-end anastomosis[6].

This study was conducted in the department of Surgery in Dhaka Medical College Hospital. The aim of this study is to determine the outcome of different modalities of treatment sigmoid volvulus and to find out a safe protocol which can be adopted in Bangladesh.

Literature review

Sigmoid volvulus is a leading cause of acute colonic obstruction in South America, Africa, Eastern Europe and Asia. It is rare in developed countries such as, The USA, UK, Japan and Australia[7]. It is more common in male and those aged over fifty years. However, the next commonly effected group is children.

Mustafa et al[8] studied on thirty-two patients to evaluate the clinical features and surgical treatment methods in patients with sigmoid volvulus. They retrospectively evaluated the demographic data of the patients, clinical features, preoperative radiological and operative findings, type of surgical procedure performed, postoperative complications, mortality and duration of hospital stay (DHS) after surgery. Surgical treatment consisted of sigmoidectomy with primary anastomosis (R&A) (n = 9, 28%), sigmoidectomy with colostomy (R&C) (n = 16, 50%) and distortion with sigmoidopexy (D&P) (n = 7, 22%). Concomitant diseases were more frequent in R&C group (n = 14, 87%) and this was statistically as compared to R&A (N = 4, 44%) (P = 0.03). Postoperative complication rate in R&C group was more frequent and DHS longer but the difference between treatment groups was not significant statistically. Two recurrences were observed in D&P group. Sigmoidectomy should be the basic principle in management of sigmoid volvulus and primary anastomosis can be performed safely in selected patients without increasing morbidity and DHS[9].

In Turan et al[10]series among the 61 patients undergoing urgent or elective operation for sigmoid volvulus, there were 17 laparotomies with only distortion, 19 resections with elective anastomosis, 6 resections with primary anastomosis and 19 resections with a Hartmann's procedure. In those cases various postoperative complications were observed. The most commonly seen complication was wound infection. In the group having emergency operations,there were 4 deaths in patients who were operatively distorted, one death in patients with anastomosis and 4 deaths in patients with Hartmann's procedure. Their results showed 9 deaths (21%) among 42 patients who underwent an emergency operation. One (5.2%) of the 19 patients died who had elective surgery because of cerebral embolus. There was no death in patients who were successfully decompressed and then followed non-operatively resection and primary anastomosis.

Objective of Hadi et al[11] series was to know the outcome of resection and end to end anastamosis with defunctioning colostomy in patients with sigmoid volvulus, operated in emergency. Patients presenting to emergency department with clinical suspicion of sigmoid volvulus, were thoroughly examined and underwent baseline and radiological investigations before surgery. Final diagnosis was made per operatively and emergency resection and end-to-end anastamosis with defunctioning colostomy were performed in all patients in casualty operation theatre. During the time period, 25 diagnosed patients with sigmoid volvulus were finally selected for the study. Seventeen patients (68%) were in their 5th and 6th decades of life. Male to female ratio was 11.5:1. In 24 operated cases (96%), the gut was viable while in one case the gut was gangrenous. The average length of stay was 7 days. Mortality was 4% (one case), which was attributed to pre-operative unstable condition and gangrenous gut at the time of surgery. They concluded that resection of sigmoid colon with primary anastamosis and a proximal defunctioning colostomy was a safer procedure in inexperienced and learning hands in emergency situations[12].

Between 1960 and 1980, 137 patients with colonic volvulus (52% caecal, 3% transverse colon, 2% splenic flexure and 43% sogmoid) were seen at Mayo Clinic[13]. Among the 59 patients with sigmoid volvulus, four (7%) had colonic infarction. Total mortality with sigmoid volvulus was seven percent. There were 71 patients with ceacal volvulus. Colonoscopic decompression was accomplished in two of these patients; in 15 (21%), gangrenous colon developed and mortality was 33%. Total mortality for cecal volvulus patients was 17%. Mortality for all forms of volvulus in patients with viable colons was 11%. Mortality for all patients with volvulus was 14%.

Sroujiehet al[14] discussed 27 patients with sigmoid volvulus treated at Jordan University Hospital (JUH) during a 15-year period. These patients represented 4.7 percent of adult patients treated for intestinal obstruction in the same period. The average age was 54.5 years and none of the patients was institutionalized. Twenty-five patients presented with acute symptoms and two had chronic symptoms. Sigmoidoscopic distortion was achieved in 15 patients. Emergency resection was required in two of these patients, for the development of gangrene a few hours after distortion I one patient and for recurrence occurred in two other patients and was managed endoscopically. Emergency surgery was performed in 10 other patients: for a failed endoscopic distortion in three patients, for ulerated and bleedingmucosaforcasting gangrene in another and as a primary treatment in six patients who were either misdiagnosed or suspected to have gangrene bowel. Elective resection was performed in 13 patients. The mortality rete was 15 percent (4/27) for the whole series and 33.3 percent (1/3) for those with gangrenous bowel.

In De series[15] betweenJanuary 1995 and December 2000, 197 patients (44.97%) were treated for sigmoid volvulus at Bankura Medical College and Hospital, Bankura, West Bengal, India. The mean age was 45.06 years and the male to female ratio was 2.07:1. The various aetiological factors, clinical features and management have been reviewed. Abdominal distension with constipation was the common clinical presentation. Straight X-ray of the abdomen suggested the diagnosis. Management included caecostomy and primary resection and anastomosis without intra-operative lavage in 196 patients and sigmoidopexy in one patient. The overall mortality rate was 1.01%. There was only recurrence in the patients who had undergone sigmoidopexy. Primary resection and anastomosis at initial presentation proved a safe operative treatment and avoided unnecessary repeated hospitalization.

Diaz-Plasenciaet al[16] evaluated 123 patients with sigmoid volvulus that underwent surgery in an attempt to identify by univariate analysis factors of prognostic value of operative mortality. The surgical procedures performed were distorted plus colopexy (n = 19), intestinal resection with primary anastomosis (n = 69) and resection plus colostomy (n = 35) with an operative death rate of 0%, 13% and 31.4% respectively (p = 0.005). The overall operative mortality rate was of 19.4%. The following parameters were evaluated: age, sex, duration of obstruction, mean arterial pressure, leukocyte count, type of peritoneal fluid, state of the bowel and surgical technique. Analysis of post-operative mortality disclosed the following factors associated with increased mortality: age older than 40 (p = 0.008), mean arterial pressure lower than 70 mmHg (p = 0.0001), presence of purulent or fecal load peritoneal fluid (p = 0.001) and evidence of gangrenous colon with perforation (p = 0.0001). There were no statistically significant differences in mortality rate with regard to sex, length of history and leukocyte count. Therefore, we emphasize the need to take into account these risk factors to better clarify appropriate therapy options.

Fifty-eight cases of colonic volvulus were reviewed by Friedman et al[17] including 30 cases of sigmoid volvulus, 27 cases of caecal volvulus and 1 of transverse colon volvulus. Decompression procedures were attempted in 31 instances of sigmoid volvulus in 27 patients and were successful 25 times (81 percent). Seven patients with sigmoid volvulus did not undergo surgery and of those, two died of unrelated causes, one was lost to follow-up, one was well and three had recurrent volvulus. Twenty-four operations were performed on 23 patients and there were three deaths (13 percent mortality). There was one recurrence in two patients who underwent simple distortion. Chronic large-bowel motility disturbances were a persistent problem in 9 of 20 (45 percent) surgical survivors. Among 27 instances of caecal volvulus, one was reduced by contrast enema and ten endoscopic attempts at decompression were unsuccessful. Twenty-six operations were done and there were four operative deaths (15 percent mortality). There were no recurrences. Large-bowel motility disorders were noted in follow-up in 3 of 22 patients (14 percent). Overall there were 10 deaths in 58 patients for a 17 percent mortality rate. These data support the importance of endoscopic decompression for sigmoid volvulus but not for caecal volvulus. Definitive treatment of both forms of volvulus should include assessment of colonic motility.

A total of 45 patients were identified in a retrospective study conducted by Theuer and Cheadle[18] and there were 17 with caecal volvulus and 29 with sigmoid volvulus (1 had both). Two-thirds of the patients were either demented, bedridden or used constipating drugs. Initial nonoperative decompression was achieved in twenty-six of twenty-nine patients with sigmoid volvulus but in only three of nine patients in which it was attempted with ceacal volvulus. Two of these recurred and sixteen of the seventeencaecal volvulus patients underwent operation. One-third of the sigmoid volvulus patients had at least one recurrent episode on the index admission. Fourteen of the twenty-nine had an operation and half of these patients died following surgery. Fifteen sigmoid volvulus patients chosen to be treated with successive non-operative treatment had no mortality. Mortality was higher following emergency (4 of 5) than elective (2 of 9) operation for sigmoid volvulus and one of three died after operation for a successfully decompressed first episode. Mortality for nonoperative reduction of an early recurrence was zero of four patients, while operative mortality for recurrence was two of seven (aa had successful preoperative deflation). There was no mortality or recurrence in four patients with ceacal volvulus treated by caecopexy alone, but all three patients' dies in which tube caecostomy was performed. Two of nine patients died following right hemicolectomy. These data suggest that if an elective operation is to be performed for sigmoid volvulus, it should be done following one or more recurrences and that nonoperative decompression can be safely performed on successive occasions.

In Edinburgh 134 patients of sigmoid volvulus were studied by Anderson and Lee[19](1981) having abdominal pain (73.9%), abdominal distention (67.7%), constipation

(47.8%), vomiting (20.1%), diarrhea (16.4%), abnormal bowel sounds (80.6%), fever (26.9%) and generalized tenderness (12.7%).

Sutcliffe[20]observed the finding in his series such as distension of abdomen in 50 cases (94%), abdominal pain 41 cases (77%), constipation 28 cases (51%), nausea and vomiting 35 cases (66%) altered bowel sound 43 cases (81%), empty rectum in 30 cases (57%), clinical evidence of dehydration 11 cases (21%) and diarrhea in 7 cases (13%).

Clinical features were also studied by authors like, Hinshaw and Carter[21] with study of 55 cases. They observed and presented their findings in cases of acute fulminating type, pain was sudden in onset and diffuse, distension was less marked and signs of prostration were present and in case of sub acute progressive type. Pain was gradual in onset, less marked and occasional cramp and abdominal distension was usually extreme and there was no sign of prostration.

Few authors have questioned the value of this clinical classification. Pool and Dunavant[22] reported that all patients presented the clinical features of complete sigmoid obstruction in different degrees of acuteness or chronocity being due to the variation in the degree of obstruction. They did not find any advantage of dividing the volvulus into different stage.

Srivasta et al[23] studied 75 cases of sigmoid volvulus in Kanpur, India from January, 1966 to March, 1970 and clinical features recorded such as abdominal Distension 75 cases (98.4%), abdominal pain in 72 cases (96%), absolute constipation in 72 cases (96%), nausea and vomiting in 27 cases (36%), dehydration in 57 cases (76%), empty rectum in 30 cases (52%), diarrhea in 3 cases (4%). Bowel sound exaggerated in 27 cases (36%).

Welch GHAND Anderson JR[24]showed a total of 50 patients aged 20-80 years, with a median age of 49 years, presented with features consistentwith large bowel obstruction. Of these, 32 had simple sigmoid volvulus and were offered sigmoid colectomy andprimary colorectal anastomosis, while 3 further patients with compound sigmoid volvulus had double resectionwith primary ileo-ileal and colorectal anastomosis. A patient with sigmoid volvulus had a Hartmann's procedure.Twelve patients had colon cancer, four had left hemicolectomy and primary colocolic anastomosis; three, sigmoidcolectomy and primary colorectal anastomosis; three, low anterior resection and primary colorectal anastomosis; onedecompressive colostomy and one, a right hemicolectomy and primary ileocolic anastomosis. The two patients'withfunctional obstruction (Ogilvie syndrome) had tube caecostomy. All resections and primary anastomosis involvingthe right colon were preceded by antegrade on-table colonic lavage. One clinical anastomotic leak occurred in alow rectal anastomosis and minor wound infection in 10 patients. Operative mortality occurred in three patientswith sigmoid volvulus.

Rennie JA[25] showed sixnumbersof patients underwent laparoscopic-assisted endoscopic sigmoidopexy for recurrent sigmoid volvulus at a mean age of 80.5 years (range, 76–83). The volvulus was decompressed endoscopically before laparoscopic adhesiolysis and detorsion of the sigmoid. Finally, the sigmoid was approximated with the anterior abdominal wall, and 2 endoscopically placed percutaneous endoscopic colostomy tubes were inserted. Later, the external component of the percutaneous endoscopic colostomy tubes was removed, and the internal parts were passed by way of the rectum. Each operation was completed successfully in a mean time of 69 minutes and with no intraoperative complication. The mean postoperative stay was 20 days (range, 4–54). At median follow-up of 10.8 months, all patients were tube free with no incidence of recurrent volvulus, inadvertent tube traction, or leak.

Bal and Boley[26] showed that sigmoid volvulus was identified in plain film X-ray of the abdomen in 34 of the 49 patients from whom they were obtained (69%).

Gurel[28]showed that in all cases plain abdominal radiograph were obtained had evidence of sigmoid volvulus.

Ballantyne[11] in his study showed that plain abdominal radiograph were diagnostic for 22 patients out of 59 patients (37%).

Taha[27] showed in his study that in all cases the path gnomic single large loop of colon arising from left iliac fossa was found in the routine erect plain abdominal radiograph.

Aims and objectives

General objective:

- To determine the outcome of different modalities treatment of sigmoid volvulus.

Specific objective:

- To find out a safe protocol which can be adopted in our country.

Rationale of this study

There are many modalities of management of sigmoid volvulus. In Dhaka Medical College Hospital there is no standard management protocol for sigmoid volvulus. In most cases conservative treatment is unsatisfactory. As flexiblesomoidoscopic or colonoscopicrelease procedure is not easily available, so laparotomy is almost always done in such case. Moreover most of the operations are performed as emergency procedure. So decision for operative procedure is not always justified by seniors. There by outcome is naturally depends on operation.

This observation prompted us to conduct this study in order to see the outcome after sigmoid volvulus treatment in different conventional methods in Dhaka Medical College Hospital.

Chapter: Two

Materials and Methods

Materials and Methods

Study design:
Descriptive case series

Place of study:
General Surgery wards of Dhaka Medical College Hospital.

Period of study:
July 2012 to December 2012.

Sample size and Sampling technique:
Total Fifty patients underwent surgery for sigmoid volvulus with fulfillment of inclusion criteria during study period. All samples were included in this study by consecutive sampling.

Inclusion criteria:
Patients admitted in surgery department of Dhaka Medical College Hospital suffering from sigmoid volvulus and treated surgically are eligible for enrollment.

Exclusion criteria:
1. Large gut obstruction due to sigmoid growth and obstruction other than volvulus.
2. Patient suffering from volvulus in any part of GIT other than sigmoid colon.
3. Sigmoid volvulus Patients with septicemia and severe co-morbid medical conditions or admitted in ICU.

Operational definition:

- **Sigmoid Volvulus:**

  Abnormal twisting of sigmoid colon along its longitudinal axis.

- **Resection- anastomosis:**

  Removal of the involved portion of the bowel and restoration of gut continuity.

- **Colostomy:**

  It is an artificial opening made in the colon to divert faeces and flatus outside the abdomen through a abdominal opening and collected in an external appliance.

Main outcome variables:

- Clinical presentation
- Treatment measures or what type of operation was performed
- Time to first oral intake
- Postoperative ileus
- Wound complications
- Anastomotic leakage
- Revesional surgery
- Length of Hospital stay

Study procedure:

All consecutive patients underwent colonic surgery fulfilling the inclusion criteria were enrolled in this study. Informed written consent was obtained from each participant. Preoperatively all patients were investigated with full blood count, plain X ray abdomen in erect posture, ultrasonography of whole abdomen, random blood sugar, blood grouping and Rh typing, blood urea, serum creatinine and serum electrolytes. Chest X ray and ECG were done also to asses the lungs and heart condition. Diagnosis was based on history, clinical examination and investigations. Treatment may include supportive and definitive. Various procedures were followed in definitive surgical treatment. Primary resection and anastomosis was done in early cases when gut was non-gangrenous and patient's general condition was good. However, Primary resection and anastomosis together with proximal diversion was done when gut was non-gangrenous and patient's general condition was not good. In late cases where gut is gangrenous and when distal part after sigmoid resection was not possible to bring out, Hartmann's procedure was done. Resection with double barrel colostomy was done in case of gangrenous gut because distal part was longer which made it easier to bring out.

Supportive treatment:

It includes nasogastric suction, intravenous fluid to correct hypovolumia and electrolytes imbalance, adequate analgesia, antibiotic administration and enema simplex when bowel sound present.

The aim of nasogastric suction is to keep the stomach empty of gas and fluid. It relieves the patient from pain and abdominal distention.

Intravenous fluids: Fluid and electrolytes imbalance invariably occur in such condition. Crystalloid solution e.g. Hartmann's solution or isotonic saline is the appropriate intravenous fluid. The amount of fluid should be justified according to the hemodynamic status of the patient. Blood transfusion is necessary if the hemoglobin level is low.

Monitoring

- Continuous catheterization and urine output should be monitored. It should be 30ml to 50ml per hour.
- Pulse, blood pressure and temperature chart should be maintained.
- Intake and output chart should be maintained. Nesogastric suction fluids have to add in output chart.
- Abdominal distention, peristaltic movement and passes of flatus and faeces should be observed.

Intravenous broad spectrum antibiotic were routinely administered preoperatively against both aerobes and anaerobes to prevent bacterial overgrowth. At every postoperative follow up patients were observed for time to first bowel movement postoperatively, time to first oral intake and sign- symptoms of development of postoperative complications like vomiting, abdominal distension, anastomotic leakage and wound complications. No follow up of the patient done after discharge from hospital. Patient's data were recorded in a prescribed Case Record Form. At the end of the study data were analyzed and the result of the study was prepared a submitted.

Study plan with flow chart:

Preparation and literature review

Protocol writing

Data collection and data analysis

Dissertation writing and submission

Work plan:

	Month 1st -3th	Month 4th	Month 5th - 11th	Month 11th - 12th
Preparation & literature review	▨			
Protocol writing		▨		
Data collection & analysis			▮	
Dissertation writing & submission				▮

Ethical measures:

Protocol was ethically reviewed and approved by the ethical review committee of BCPS. Institutional clearance was obtained from appropriate authority of Dhaka Medical College Hospital, Dhaka. Detailed study related information was read out and explained from a printed hand out. All aspect including confidentiality and right not be participated would be duly considered.

Methods of data processing and statistical analyses:

All the relevant data were compiled on a master chart first. Statistical analysis of the results is obtained by using windows based computer software. The continuous data are expressed as mean ± SD. The categorical data are expressed as number and percentage. The results are presented in tables and diagrams.

Chapter: Three

Results

Results

This study was conducted to observe the results after performing of operation for sigmoid volvulus by different modalities. Total fifty patients were included in this study. The findings of the study are presented here in detail.

Table 3.1 Distribution of patient by age(n=50)

Age of patient in yrs	Number of patients	Percentage (%)
20-30	03	06
31-40	09	18
41-50	11	22
51-60	15	30
61-70	12	24

Mean $\pm$ Standard deviation= 54.98 $\pm$ 11.27

Table 3.1 shows that the highest number (15 cases; 30%) of the patients are in the age group of 51-60 years. The mean age of the patients is 54.98 years (SD$\pm$ 11.27). 12 (24%) patients were found in 61-70 years age groups. No patient was found in below 20 years.

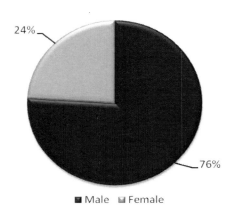

Figure 3.1 Distribution of patients by gender

Figure 3.1 shows that, most of the patients were male (38 cases; 76%).12 (24%)patients were female. Male to female ratio was 3.17:1.

Table 3.2 Presenting features:

Complaints	Frequency	Percentage (%)
Abdominal pain	43	86
Absolute constipation	50	100
Abdominal distention	50	100
Nausea and Vomiting	24	48
Dehydration	23	46
Respiratory Distress	27	54
Fever	11	22
H/O Chronic Constipation	13	26
First attack		
Recurrent history of intestinal obstruction		
History and sign of previous surgery (abdominal)		

Table 3.2 shows that, all the patients (100%) had the complaints of failure to pass stool or flatus andabdominal distention. Abdominal pain was complained by 43 (86%) patients. However, respiratory distress, Nausea and vomiting, dehydration was observed in about 50% of the patients.

Table 3.3: Distribution of patients by Operative procedure (n = 50)

Type of operation	Frequency(Number)	Percentage (%)
Resection and primary anastomosis	16	32
Hartmann's procedure	21	42
Resection and double barrel colostomy	06	12
Resection and primary anastomosis with proximal colostomy	07	14
Total	50	100

Table 3.3 shows that commonly performed operation was Hartmann's Operation (42%), Second common operation was performed Resection and primary anastomosis(32%). The other procedures were Resection and primary anastomosis with proximal colostomy (14%) and Resection with double barrel colostomy (12%).

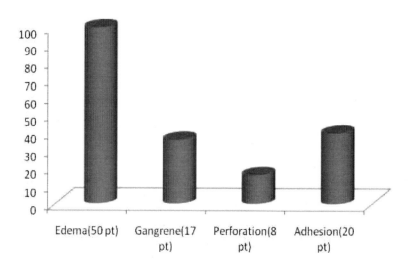

Fig. 3.2: Operative findings of the patients

Fig. 3.2 shows that during operation the gut condition of the all patients (100%) found edematous. In 40% patients adhesions was found. Gangrene was found in 34% patients and Perforation in 16%.

29

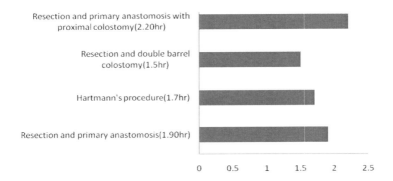

Fig. 3.3: Duration of operation (Mean ± SD=1.83±0.39 (hr)

Fig. 3.3 shows that among the four procedures, resection and primary anastomosis with proximal colostomy took the highest operative hour (2.20 hr) whereas Resection and double barrel colostomy took the lowest operative hour(1.50 hr). The mean operation hour was 1.83 hr.

Table 3.4: Time to first bowel movement postoperatively

Time to bowel movement	Number of patient	Percentage (%)
< 24 hours	0	0
24 to 48 hours	18	36
48 to 72 hours	26	52
>72 hours	06	12
Total	50	100

Table 3.4shows that 26 patients (52%) moved their bowel postoperatively within 48 to 72 hours and 24 patients (36%) moved bowel within 24 to 48 hours. Small number of patients 6 (12%) out of 50, moved their bowel after 72 hours.

Table 3.5 Post operative complications

3.5 a Resection and primary anastomosis (Total patient = 16)

Complications	Frequency	Percentage (%)
Wound complication (Infection, dehiscence and burst abdomen)	05	31.25
Febrile illness	06	37.5
Anastomotic leakage	01	6.25
Electrolytes imbalance	02	12.5
Post operative ileus	01	6.25
Revisional surgery (Laparotomy)	01	6.25
Death	01	6.25

Out of 16 patients, who underwent operation of Resection and primary anastomosis (Table 3.5 a), highest numbers of patients (37.5%) were suffered from febrile illness followed by wound complication *i.e.* infection, dehiscence and burst abdomen (31.25%).

3.5 b: Hartmann's procedure (Total patient = 21)

Complications	Frequency	Percentage (%)
Wound complication (Infection, dehiscence and burst abdomen)	08	38.10
Febrile illness	10	47.62
Electrolytes imbalance	04	19.05
Post operative ileus	02	9.52
Revisional surgery (Laparotomy)	01	4.76
Death	03	14.29

In Hartmann's procedure (Table 3.5 b), out of 21 patients, highest numbers of patients (47.62%) were suffered from febrile illness followed by wound complication *i.e.* infection, dehiscence and burst abdomen (38.10%).

Complications	Frequency	Percentage (%)
Wound complication (Infection, dehiscence and burst abdomen)	02	33.33
Febrile illness	02	33.33
Electrolytes imbalance	01	16.67
Post operative ileus	01	16.67
Revisional surgery (Laparotomy)	00	00
Death	01	16.67

3.5 c: Resection and double barrel colostomy (Total patient = 06)

In Resection and double barrel colostomy (Table 3.5 c), among all the complications revisional surgery (Laparotomy) was absent. Patients with wound complication *i.e.* infection, dehiscence and burst abdomen followed by febrile illness were found higher (33.33%) whereas electrolytes imbalance, post operative ileus were found lower (16.67%). Only one patient (16.67%) was succumbed to death.

3.5 d: Resection and primary anastomosis with proximal colostomy (Total patient = 07)

Complications	Frequency	Percentage (%)
Wound complication (Infection, dehiscence and burst abdomen)	03	42.86
Febrile illness	03	42.86
Anastomotic leakage	00	00
Electrolytes imbalance	01	14.29
Post operative ileus	01	14.29
Revisional surgery (Laparotomy)	00	00
Death	01	14.29

Out of 07 patients, who underwent operation of Resection and primary anastomosis (Table 3.5 d) with proximal colostomy, anastomotic leakage and revisional surgery complications were absent among all the patients. In one hand, highest numbers of patients *i.e.* three (42.86%) were suffered from wound complication *i.e.* infection, dehiscence and burst abdomen followed by febrile illness.

Table 3.6: Duration of hospital stay

Length of hospital stay	Number of patient	Percentage (%)
Less than 7 days	02	04
7 to 10 days	27	54
More than 10 days	16	32
Death	05	10
Total	50	100

Mean length of postoperative hospital stay 10.33days (SD$\pm$ 3.99)

Table 3.6 shows that, most of the patients were discharged from the hospital within 7 to 10 days. Only 2 patients (4%) were discharged before 7 days whereas 32% patient stayed in the hospital more than 10 days.5 patients (10%)succumbed to death.

Chapter: Four

Discussion

Discussion

Sigmoid volvulus is a leading cause of acute colonic obstruction in South America, Africa, Eastern Europe and Asia. It is the most common part of the gastrointestinal tract to be affected by volvulus and accounts for up to 10% of all cases of intestinal obstruction. Once the diagnosis of sigmoid volvulus is confirmed, treatment must be immediate, as delay means more likelihood of bowel wall ischemia and gangrene. Up to 80% of people with this condition die from gangrene if intervention is delayed.

The treatment of sigmoid volvulus has evolved over the past decades from one requiring immediate surgical correction, which carries a high mortality, to one of immediate sigmoidoscopic decompression and elective surgery with its attendant lower mortality. More recently the use of the flexible sigmoidoscope or colonoscope provides a further weapon in the armamentarium of the surgeon attempting non operative reduction of the sigmoid loop. The treatment of sigmoid volvulus is a complex procedure. Many studies have shown that patient with early presentation where laparoscopic intervention can be done, the outcome is better.

The currently accepted surgical procedures for sigmoid volvulus include sigmoid resection with primary anastomosis and resection & Hartman procedure. The other methods are Paul-Mikulicz procedure, sigmoidopexy, mesosigmoidopexy, extraperitonealization of sigmoid colon, mesenteropexy, laparoscopic fixation and percutaneous endoscopic colopexy using colonscopy.

This study was conducted over 50 admitted patients in General Surgery wards of Dhaka Medical College Hospital, who underwent emergency surgery after proper resuscitation.

In the present study it was observed that, among the patients who were undertaken for sigmoid volvulus operationare usually 20 to 70 years old. Among these 30 (60%)patients belonged to 51 to 60 years old followed by 61 to 70 years old (24%).On the other hand,the lowest group found in 20 to 30 year'sage group (6%). Considering all the patients, the average age range was 54.98 years (Table 3.1). Same result was found in a study conducted by Md Z. Haq (1996)[35] and Md. R. Islam (2008)[36].Similarly, N.A Baloch and M.A. Baloch (2004) reported an average age range of 56.1 years in his study. It was also found that, among all the patients 76% were male and only 24% were female[29](Fig 3.1). It could be said that, male patient suffer a lot from this disease.Md Z. Haq (1996)[35] and Md. R. Islam (2008)[36], also found almost same male and female ratio.

All of the patients, who were admitted to the hospital, came with the complaints of abdominal distension and failure to pass stool or flatus. Most prioritizing fact is that, 86% of the patients were suffering from abdominal pain whereas 100% suffered from the same in a study conducted by Md Z. Haq (1996)[35] and Md. R. Islam (2008)[36].Almost 50% of the patients were suffered from nausea, vomiting, dehydration and respiratory distress. Minority of the patients were suffered from fever (22%) and history of chronic constipation (26%) (Table 3.2). Gray J. Arnold et al (1973) also found a close history where 87% of the patient suffered from abdominal pain and distension, 35% from nausea and vomiting, 27% from constipation[30].

In the current study, it was found that all the patients were undertaken into emergency operation. Among those patients, 42% were operated through Hartmann's procedure whereas only 12% were operated through resection and double barrel colostomy. From the rest of the patients, 32% were operated through resection and primary anastomosis and 14% were through resection and primary anastomosis with proximalcolostomy (Table 3.3).

After laparotomy, it was found that sigmoid colon edema was present in all the patients. Adhesion was found in 40% of the patient's. In 34 % of the patient, sigmoid colon was gangrenous whereas sigmoid colon was perforated in 16% of the patient (Fig. 3.2). In a study in Bangladesh, sigmoid colon was gangrenous in 28% patients (Md Z. Haq, 1996)[35]. However, the reason of higher percentage in this study is due to delayed admission in hospital.

This study showed that, among all the procedures, resection and primary anastomosis with proximal colostomy was time consuming as it took 2.2 hours. Resection and double barrel colostomy was the economical one as it took only 1.50 hours. Mean operational time was 1.83 hours(Fig.3.3).

In the present study, bowel moved within 48 to 72 hours in almost 52% of the patient. 12% of the patient took more than 72 hours (Table 3.4). Similar outcome was also found in a study conducted by Aslam V. (2008)[31].

While observing post operative complications,among the four procedures performed, wound complication was found in higher percentage (42.86%) in resection and primary anastomosis with proximal colostomy (Table 3.5 d). Lower percentage (31.25%) was found in resection and primary anastomosis (Table 3.5 a) whereas percentage was higher (41.2) in a study conducted by Dr. Md. R. Islam (2008)[36]. The reason could be use of broad spectrum antibiotics in proper time and also meticulous operation. Higher percentage (47.62%) of febrile illness was found in Hartmann's procedure (Table 3.5 b) whereas lower percentage (33.33%) was found in resection and double barrel colostomy (Table 3.7). Electrolytes imbalance was higher (19.05%) in Hartmann's procedure (Table 3.5 b) whereas lower (12.5%) in resection and primary anastomosis (Table 3.5 a).In resection and primary anastomosis, anastomotic leakage was 6.25% in this study while 8% was found in Md. R. Islam's (2008)[36]study. Resection and double barrel colostomy (Table 3.5 c) showed higher percentage (16.67%) of postoperative ileus while resection and primary anastomosis (Table 3.5 a) showed the lower percentage (12.5%).

Revisional surgery was found higher (6.25%) in resection and primary anastomosis while no revisional surgery was needed in resection and double barrel colostomy and in resection and primary anastomosis with proximal colostomy. Death rate was high (16.67%) in resection and double barrel colostomy and low in resection and primary anastomosis (6.25%). In a study conducted by Md Z. Haq (1996)[35]death rate was found almost same in resection and primary anastomosis (5.54 %). The average hospital stay found in this study was 10.33 days (Table 3.6).

In a study with resection and primary anastomosis procedure, among the patient, the percentage of wound infection, death and hospital stay was 18.2%, 4.5% and 12 days respectively (N A. Baloch and M A. Baloch, 2008)[29].However, Aslam V. et al (2008) reported in one stage resection method that, among the patient, the rate of mortality was 30 to 50%, paralytic ileus 22%, wound infection 14% respectively[31]. According to Martin G. et al (1977), death rate was 6% in primary resection and anastomosis procedure while 6% death rate in Paul Mikulitz operation[32].

AZ Sule and A. Ajibade (2011), conducted a similar study and reported that, wound infection and death rate was 16% and 5.25%. In Hartmann's procedure death rate was 73% and mean hospital stay was 7 to 25 days[33].

Qzdemir et al (2012) suggested that wound infection and anastomotic leakage was 36.15% and 3.85% in primary resection and anastomosis procedure where mean hospital stay was 8.6 days[34].

From this study together with several literature reviews as mentioned earlier, it was found that among all the procedure, in Resection and primary anastomosis the death rate, wound complication, electrolyte imbalance, post operative ileus was the lowest (Table 3.5 a) which mainly determines the early recovery of a patient. Moreover, further operation for gut restoration is not needed in this procedure that reduces patients' morbidity.

Conclusion

This study concluded that, in a country like Bangladesh flexible Colonoscopic or Sigdoscopic reduction is not easily available in everywhere. Under these circumstances, Resection and Primary anastomosis could be the most convenient and promising for both patient and surgeon if gut condition is favourable.It could also lighten the burden on national economy as well as reduce the post operative morbidity of the patient.

Limitations of the study:

1. The sample size was relatively small.
2. Duration of the study was short.
3. The long term complications of the operative procedure could not be assessed.
4. Only important postoperative complications were observed.
5. Only four operative procedures were used in the present study apart from the advanced procedure due to lack of technological support

Suggestions for further study:

Further study must be needed combining large sample size using more and long term complications. Most challenging could be the use of advanced procedure (Flexible Sigmoidoscopic or Colonoscopic reduction) if advanced technological support is available.

References cited

1. Raveenthiran V, Madiba TE, AtamanalpSS,et al; Volvulus of the sigmoid colon.Colorectal Dis.2010 Jul;12(7 Online):e1-17.Epub 2010 Mar 10.(abstract)

2. Martinez AD, Yanez LJ, Souto R. Indication and results of endoscopic management of sigmoid volvulus, Rev EspEnferm Dig. 2003; 95: 538-539.

3. Dr.Sarah Jarvis'Patient.co.uk-Trusted medical information and support, 2011 Mar 28; 01:01-06.

4. Dr. Swapan Kumar Biswas, Dr. JC Saha, Dr. AZMMostaqueHossain. Faridpur Medical College Journal 2009 Jan; 4(1): 01-03.

5. UpToDate, Inc. All rights reserved. 2012; Support Tag: [ecapp1104p.utd.com-180.234.67.239-4E058D1F0C-14]

6. Garth H.Ballantyne. Practice limited to laparoscopic surgery 2010 Sep: 01-06.

7. Lau KCN, Miller BJ, Schache DJ, Cohen JR. Astudy of large-bowel volvulus in urban Australia. Can J Surg2006; 49: 203-207.

8. Mustafa NA, Yucel Y, Turkyilmaz S, surgical treatment of the sigmoid volvulus. ActaChirBelg 2005; 105: 365-368.

9. Madiba TE and Thomson SR. The management of sigmoid volvulus. J R CollSurgEdinb April 2000; 45:74-80.

10. Turan M, Sen M, Karadayi K, Koyuncu A, Topcu O, Yildirir C et al. our sigmoid colon volvulus ecperience and benefits of colonscope in detortion process. Rev EspEnferm Dig (Madrid) 2004; 96: 32-35.

11. Hadi A, Khan M, Shah SMA, Bangash A. Emregency management of sigmoid volvulus: experience of Lady Reading Hospital Peshawar. J Postgrad Medn Inst 2006; 20: 82-5.

12. OncuM,PiskinB,Calik A, et al. Volvulus of sigmoid colon. S Afr J Surg 1991; 29:48-49.

13. Ballantyne GH. Review of sigmoid volvulus: history and results of treatment. Dis Colon Rectum 1982; 25: 494-501.

14. Sroujieh AS, Farah Gr, Jabaiti SK, el-Muhtaseb HH, Qudah MS, Abu-Khalaf MM, Volvulus of the sigmoid colon in Jordan. Dis Colon Rectum 1992; 35: 64-8.

15. De U. Sigmoid volvulus in rural Bengal. Trop Doct. 2002 Apr; 32(2): 80-2.

16. Diaz-Plasencia J, Sanchez C, Bardales M, Rebaza H, Calipuy W. Operative mortality in sigmoid volvulus. RevGastroenterol Peru 1993; 13: 37-44.

17. Friedman JD, Odland MD, Bubrick MP, Experience with colonic volvulus. Dis Colon Rectum 1989; 32: 409-16.

18. Theuer C, Cheadle WG, Volvulus of the colon. Am Surg. 1999; 57: 145-50.

19. Anderson JR, Lee D. The management of acute sigmoid volvulus. Br J Surg 2000; 68: 117-120.

20. Sutcliffe. Volvulus of sigmoid colon.Br. J. Sung 1968; 55: 903-10

21. Hinshaw DB, Carter R. Surgical management of acute sigmoid volvulus. Annuls of Surgery 1957; 146: 52-60.

22. Pool RM, Dunavant WD. Volvulus of the sigmoid colon. Ann Surg 1951; 133: 719-26.

23.Srivastava RD, Rajpur VS, Gewal. Volvulus of the sigmoid colon. J. Surg. Sci. 1972; 8: 81-87.

24. Welch GH, Anderson JR. Acute volvulus of sigmoid colon. World J.Surg 1987; 11:258-62.

25. RennieJA. Sigmoid volvulus. Journal of the Royal Society of Medicine 1979; 72: 654-656.

26. Bal MP, Boley SJ. Sigmoid volvulus in elderly patients. American Journal of Surgery 1986; 151:71-75.

27. Taha SE, Suleiman SI. Volvulus of the sigmoid colon in the Gezira. British Journal of Surgery 1980; 67: 433-435.

28. Gurel M, Alic B. Intra-operative colon irrigation in the treatment of acute sigmoid volvulus. British Journal of Surgery 1989; 176: 957-958.

29. N A. Baloch, M A. Baloch. Resection and Primary anastomosis.Pakistan Journal of Surrrgery 2008; 24(2): 1-3.

30. Gray J. Arnold, Francies, Nance. Volvulus of the sigmoid colon. Ann. Surg. May 1973; 171: 527-531.

31. ViqarAslam, Mohammad Abed Khan, Mohammad Bilal Zaiulabidin. One stage Resection of Sigmoid Volvulus; an experience of 50 cases. JPMI 2008; 22(3): 225-228.

32. Martin G, Wertkin, MD Arthur, Aufes, Jr. Md. Management of volvulus of colon. Department of Surgery, Mount Sinai School of Medicine of the City University of Newyork 1977; 21(1): 1-2.

33. A. Z. Sule, A. Ajibade. Adult large bowel obstruction: A review of clinical experience. Annuals of African Medicine 2011; 10(1): 45-50.

34. OzdemirSuleyman, Md. Aslar A. Kassaf, Kuzu M. Ayhan. Sigmoid volvulus: Long term clinical outcome and review of the literature. SAJS 2012; 50(1): 9.

35. Md. ZahurulHaq. Outcome of emergency resection of sigmoid volvulus (dissertation-BCPS).Depatment of Surgery, IPGMR 1996.

36. Md. Rafiqul Islam. Study of different modalities of treatment of sigmoid volvulus (dissertation-BCPS). Department of Surgery, Dhaka Medical College Hospital 2008.

Appendices

Appendix A:

DATA COLLECTION SHEET

1. Particulars of the patient:

Name: Sex: M/F

Age: Religion:

Marital status: Occupation:

Address: Phone No:

2.Hospital reference:

Surgery Unit: Reg. no:

Ward/Cabin: Date of admission:

Bed no: Date of examination:

Date of operation: Date of discharge:

3. History:

a) Presenting complaints: b) History of present illness:

c)History of past illness: d) Drug history:

e)Treatment history: f) Socio economic history:

g)Personal history: h) Nicotine use-Y/N

4.Physical examination:

General examination:

    a) Appearance: b) Body built: c) Decubitus:
    d) Nutritional status: e) Anaemia: f) Jaundice:
    g) Cyanosis: h) Edema: i) Dehydration:
    j)   Enlarged lymph node: k) Engorged vein: l) Pulse:
    m) BP: n) Resp rate: 0) Temp:

Local examination:

- a) Inspection:
- b) Percussion:

b) Palpation:
d) Auscultation:

DRE:
Other systemic examination:
- a) Alimentary system:
- c) Cardiovascular system:
- e) Musculoskeletal system:

b) Respiratory system:
d) Genitourinary system:
f) Nervous system:

Pre-operative investigation:
Blood for-
TC-/mm3
DC-
N:L:M:E:B:
ESR:mm in 1sthr,Hb%-
RBS:
Blood grouping and Rh typing:

Serum creatinine-
Serum electrolytes-
Urine RME:
Plain X-ray abdomen:
X-ray chest PA view:
USG of whole abdomen:

CT scan of the abdomen:
Proctoscopy/Sigmoidoscopy:
Ba enema:

Operation note:
Date and time:
Indication:
Anaesthesia:
Incision:
Findings:
Procedure:
Post operative complication:
Revisional surgery: Date of first follow up:

APPENDIX -B

Informed Written Consent

1. **Protocol ID :**
2. **Title of the study:**Outcome of Different Modalities Treatment of Sigmoid Volvulus: A Study of Fifty Cases
3. **Investigator's name:**Dr.Pradip Kumar Nath
4. **Institution/ Organisation:**Dhaka Medical College Hospital.
5. **Purpose of the study:**Treatment of sigmoid volvulus is a complex procedure. There are different types of treatment modalities which are traditionally practiced.The present study is attempted to observe the outcome of different operative treatments. This study will also find out the most convenient, economic and less morbid procedure.
6. **Selection of the participant:**As your age is above 20 years and you undergone colonic surgery as an emergency operation, you can participate in our study according to selection criteria.
7. **Expectation from and involvement of the participant:**If you agree to participate in this study you will be asked some questions and you will be observed post operatively during the period of your hospital stay. But you will not be subjected to any kind of intervention of your treatment by this study.
8. **Risk and benefits:**You have no risk if you participate in this study rather if any complication arises during your treatment period that can be promptly detected and solved by this study. You will not get any financial support if you participate in this study.
9. **Privacy, anonymity and confidentiality:**Information gathered from this study will be used only for the purpose of research. The name of the participants and their personal information will remain confidential.
10. **Right to withdraw:**If you wish you have the right to withdraw from this study at any point of time.

If you agree to our proposal of enrolling you / your patient in our study, please indicate that by putting your signature or your left thumb impression at the specified space below.
Thank you for your cooperation.

_____
Signature or left thumb impression of the participant

_____   _____
Signature or left thumb impression of a witness   Signature of the investigator

Date: …………………………..

APPENDIX-C

wjwLZ m¤§wZcÎ

1. প্রটোকলআইডি :
2. গবেষণারটাইটেল: Outcome of different modalities treatment of Sigmoid Volvulus; A study of 50 cases.
3. গবেষকেরনাম :ডাঃ প্রদীপ কুমার নাখ।
4. হাসপাতাল :ঢাকামেডিকেলকলেজহাসপাতাল।
5. গবেষনারউদ্দেশ্য :সিগময়েড ভলভুলাস এর চিকিৎসা একটি জটিল প্রক্রিয়া। গতানুগতিক বিবিধ পদ্ধতি রয়েছে এর চিকিৎসার জন্য। এই গবেষণার উদ্দেশ্য হল বিভিন্ন অপারেশন পদ্ধতির পরবর্তী সময়ে রোগীর কি ধরনের উন্নতি বা জটিলতা হয় তা পরিলক্ষিত করা। এই গবেষণার আরও উদ্দেশ্য হল কোন পদ্ধতিটি তুলনামুলক নিরাপদ এবং আমাদের দেশের জন্য মান সম্পন্ন ও গ্রহণযোগ্য হয়।
6. অংশগ্রহণকারীনিবার্চন :যেহেতুআপনারবয়স ২০ বছরেরউপরেএবং আপনার এই রোগের জন্য অপারেশনকরাহবে,অতএবউক্তগবেষণারনিয়মঅনুযায়ীআপনিএতেঅংশগ্রহনকরতেপারবেন।
7. অংশগ্রহণকারীরকায়র্প্রণালী :আপনিযদিএইগবেষণায়অংগগ্রহনকরেনতাহলেআপনাকেকিছুপূবনির্ধারিতপ্রশ্নকরাহবেএবংঅপারেশরআগেওপরেআপনাকেকয়েকবারপরীক্ষাওপযবেক্ষনকরেপ্রয়জনীয়তথ্যসংগ্রহকরাহবে।তবেআপনারচিকিৎসাপদ্ধতিতেহস্তক্ষেপকরাহবেনা।
8. ঝুঁকিএবংসুবিধা :এইগবেষণায়আপনারকোনঝুঁকিনেইবরংচিকিৎসাকালীনসময়েকোনপ্রকারজটিলতাদেখাদিলেতাদ্রুতলির্ণয়ওলিরাময়করাসম্ভব। এইগবেষণায়অংগগ্রহনেরজন্যআপনাকেকোনপ্রকারআর্থিকসুবিধাদেয়াহবেনা।
9. গোপনীয়তারক্ষা :সংগৃহীততথ্যাদিকেবলগবেষণারকাজেব্যবহৃতহবে।অংশগ্রহণকারীরনামওব্যাক্তিগততথ্যাদিপ্রকাশকরাহবেনা।
10. গবেষণাথেকেসরিয়েনেওয়ারক্ষমতা :আপনিযদিসিদ্ধান্তনেনযেআপনিএইগবেষণায়থাকবেননাতাহলেআপনিযেকোনসময়এইগবেষণাথেকেলিজেকেসরিয়েলিতেপারবেন।

আপনিযদিউপবোল্লিখিতপ্রস্তাবমেনেআপনাকে/ আপনারেরোগীকেআমারগবেষণারঅন্তর্ভুক্তকরতেচান,তাহলেঅনুগ্রহপূবর্কলিেচেনিধার্রিতস্থানেআপনারস্বাক্ষর/ বামহাতেরবৃদ্ধাসুলিরছাপপ্রদানকরুন।

আপনারসহায়তারজন্যধন্যবাদ।

--   ---

অংশগ্রহণকারীরস্বাক্ষর/বামহাতেরবৃদ্ধাসুলিরছাপস্বাক্ষরীরস্বাক্ষর/বামহাতেরবৃদ্ধাসুলিরছাপ

গবেষকেরস্বাক্ষর.......................

তারিখ :……….............

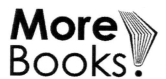
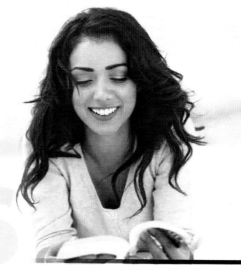
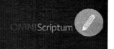

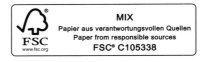

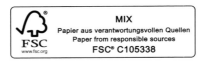

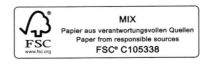